**Definition of Lactation:**

**Lactation** is the secretion of milk from the <u>breast</u> and the period of time that a **mother,** and her baby.

## Hormones responsible about lactation:

**At the week of 24 of pregnancy, hormones stimulate the growth the duct sytem in the breast**

<u>Progesterone</u>

It stimulates the size of <u>alveoli</u> and lobes; before labour high levels of progesterone suppresses lactation. After labor there is sudden drop in progesterone levels drop this stimulate milk production.

<u>Estrogen:</u>

Estrogen stimulate duct system to grow , and sudden drop in its level following labour induce milk production. It remain at low level during period of lactation.

## Prolactin:

It increases growth of the alveoli, and differentiation of duct system. prolactin maintains junctions of the ductal epithelium and regulating milk production by osmotic balance. It also increases growth factor levels (IGF-1), and lipid metabolism in preparation for milk.

## ACTH (adreno-cortico-tropic hormone) and glucocorticoids:

ACTH is structurally similar to prolactin. Glucocorticoids maintenances the tight junctions.

## TSH

It is lactation induction hormone ,and its levels are increased during pregnancy.

## Oxytocin

Oxytocin is essential for the *milk ejection reflex*.

## Human placental lactogen (HPL):

the placenta releases large amounts of HPL the second month of pregnancy. This hormone appears to be helpful in breast, nipple, and areola maturation .

Other hormons:

Follicle stimulating hormone (FSH)

Luteinizing hormone (LH)

**Factors are necessary to maintain the milk supply:**

**1-Neuro-Endrocrine**

- Intact neuro-hormonal pathways
- Suckling, breast stimulation,

**2- Autocrine**

**3- Milk Removal**

**Endocrine (Hormonal) Control of Milk Synthesis — Lactogenesis I & II**

During pregnancy and the first few days postpartum, the *endocrine control system* control milk supply.

Lacto genesis I:

Colostrums were made about mid pregnancy.

(Lactogenesis II):

Milk will increase in volume around 30-40 hours after birth.

At the end of pregnancy, the breasts are making colostrums, due to high levels of progesterone milk secretion will inhibited. After delivery of the placenta there is sudden drop in progesterone/estrogen/HPL levels. This rapid withdrawal of progesterone in the presence of high prolactin levels start Lacto genesis II (profuse milk production. After 50-73 hours (2-3 days) after birth mothers usually begin feeling increased breast fullness (the sensation of breast engorgement)

**Maintenance of milk supply:**

**Autocrine (Local) Control of Milk Synthesis ( Lactogenesis III).** This Maintenance stage of milk production is also called local control system. In the maintenance stage, milk removal is controlling milk synthesis. Milk removal is determined by baby's hunger. Hormonal problems can still delay milk supply. Under normal conditions the breasts will continue to make milk for ever as long as milk removal continues.

## Milk Ejection Response (Let-down)

The tension in the breast is persistent when the milk does not go off of the breast. The milk ejection response (MER) is the action illicit by oxytocin on the smooth muscle of each alveolus. Contraction of the alveoli vigorously push the milk into the ducts to the nipple and finally to the infant. As he baby continues to suck, additional MER's take place. In the early days of breast lactation, five to eight minutes is needed for the first let-down to occur. Oxytocin, as prolactin, is released in waves. It has a very short life span in maternal serum. The first wave begins before the baby is put to breast (triggered emotionally by mother thinking to feed or hearing infant crying). Following release is in response to nipple stretching uterine contraction in response to Oxitocin may cause pain for the mothers. let down sensation usually started after the first week or two.

Factors affecting milk dynamics:

- Gestational age at birth (preterm and full term).
- Stage of lactation. (colustrums and mature milk).
- During lactation (fore milk and hind milk).

**Benefits of breast feeding:**

**Breast feeding has many benefits:**

**1- Infants.**

**2- Mothers.**

**3- Family.**

**4Community.**

## Benefits of breast feeding for infants:

**Importance of colostrums:**

1- Antibody rich protect fro infection, and allargy.

2- Many white cells protect against infection.

3- Purgative protect against jaundice.

4- Growth factor help intestine to mature and  prevent intolerance.

5- Rich in vitamin A protect against eye disorders.

6- The colostrum acts as a laxative cleaning the infant's stomach.

## Benefits of breast milk for thr infants:

**1-Infants nutrition:**

- It contains all the needed nutrients for the infant first 6 months in optimum magnitude, and adequate quantities.
- It promotes adequate growth and development
- It is sterile, and clean.
- Easy to digest, and to absorb.
- Breast milk provides adequate water for hydration.

2. Protect infant from infection.

It contains antibodies especially against diarrhoea and respiratory infections.

3-Adequate  temperature and always ready.

4-It protects against allergies.

5-It contains enough water for the baby's needs (87% of water and minerals).

6-It helps jaw and teeth development. Suckling develops facial muscles

7-Psychomotor, emotional and social development of the infant due to frequent skin-to-skin contact between mother and infant.

7- Intelligence development.

9-Bonds Mother and Child.it decreases **the rate of** infant abandonment.

10 -Enhance vaccine response.

11-Prevents diseases in adult hood.
AIDS
Allergies
Appendix
Arthritis

Asthma

Diabetes Mellitus

Eczema

Gastroesophageal Reflex

Haemophilus Influenza

Obesity

Leukemia

Meningitis

Multiple Sclerosis

ecrotizing Enternal Colitis (NEC)

Sudden Infant Death Syndrome (SIDS)

**Benefits of breast milk for pre matures:**

- o It shortens length of hospital stay.
- o Reduces hospital costs.
- o Helps brainstem maturation.
- o Reduces the risk of life-threatening disease of the gastrointestinal system and other infectious diseases.

**Benefits of Breastfeeding for the Mother:**

1- Oxytocine sitmulates uterine contractions, and restoration of its normal size after labour.

2- Effective methods of contraception ,it promots amenorrhea may be for 6 months.

3- Breast milk production is stimulated when breast feeding started immediately after birth.

4- It prevents breast engorgement.

5- It prevents work and time for preparation of bottle feeding.

6- Prevents premenopausal breast and ovarian cancers.

7- Psychological bond between mother and her baby,

**Benefits of Breastfeeding for the Family:**

1- Financially ,it decreases expenses for buying infant formula.

2- It decreases medical expenses for frequent illiness.

3- It decreases emotional disturbances associated with baby illieness.

4- Births are spaced because it act contraception.

**Benefits of Breastfeeding for the Community.**

1. Not importing infant formula.

2. Healthy individuals.

3. Less national exepense on medical support.

4. Protect enviorement

**Anesthesia and breast lactation:**

Anesthesia can interfere either direct or indirect:

**Direct effects of anesthesia on breast lactation:**

Anesthesia can interfere with lactation in three stages:

1- Anesthesia during labor, and cesarean section.
It can affect initiation of breast lactation, and delay or prevent colostrums.

## Advantages of general anesthesia during labor and cesarean section:

- General anesthesia can be induced rapidly, and this is very helpful if an emergency cesarean section is mandatory.
- This can be administered without requiring a change in position.
- General anesthesia always provides adequate pain relief.
- When regional anesthesia is contraindicated, when patient has back surgery or has back deformities. Some patients with brain tumors or increased intracranial pressure may not be able to receive an epidural or spinal anesthetic.

**The risks associated with general anesthesia can be life threatening and include:**

**Disadventages:**

1. Complete recovery of the mothers and be able for nursing her baby

2. Respiratory depression of the neonate

3. Sleepy newborn, make the newborn initiates breast feeding,and get the thr benefit of colustrum.

4. Toxic effects of anesthetics on the newborn.

### General anesthesia and vaginal delivery.

General anesthesia may be used to protect the mother or baby in emergency situations, such as:

- difficult forceps

- Breech presentation.

- Shoulder dystocia .

- internal cephalic version (manipulation of the fetus into a head-first presentation while still in the uterus

- Delivery a second twin.

  2- Anesthesia in lactating mothers.

  3- Post operative analgesia.

## Factors affect Drug Entry into Human Milk:

The amount of drug excreted into milk depends on:

**Drugs pharmacokinetics:**

1) The lipid solubility of the drug,

2) The molecular size of the drug,

3) The blood level attained in the maternal circulation,

4) Protein binding in the maternal circulation,

5) Oral bioavailability in the infant.

6) The half-life in the maternal and infant's plasma compartments.

## Drugs pharmacdynamics:

## Early post partum after labor and cesarean section

Usually drugs enter milk during the neonatal period more than in mature milk by two major mechanisms.

**1-Diffusion method.**

**2-Secretory method.**

Drugs pass from the maternal plasma compartment through the capillary walls into the alveolar cell lining the milk buds. They have to pass through both walls of the alveolar cells to infiltrate milk in the first 4 to 10 days lactation, large differences between alveolar cells be present. These differences allow better access for most drugs, many immunoglobulins, maternal lymphocytes, and other maternal proteins to the milk. Afterward the first week, the alveolar cells distend, later closing the intracellular gaps and limiting entrance to the milk.

### 3-Maternal Plasma Level:

Mother's plasma level is the most important determinant factor for drug diffusion into milk. More or less without exclusion, as the plasma level of the drugs in the mother's plasma starts to rise, the concentration in milk begins its rise as well. Drugs enter milk, and, leave milk as a role of the decreased; the milk level almost immediately follows.

### 4- Ion Trapping:

Ion trapping means, drugs become ion trapped in milk, due to

- **The lower pH of human milk:**
  The physicochemical composition of the drug changes, and inhibits its perfusion reverse into the maternal circulation.
- Specialized transport systems that "push" substances into milk Trapping can also occur. This is important in weakly basic drugs (barbiturates. So the drug may concentrate in milk at high milk/plasma ratios. ·

## Protein Binding and Lipophilicity:

- **lipid solubility**.

Drugs that are very lipid soluble, penetrate milk in higher concentrations as opioids . Especially drugs act in the central nervous system (CNS). CNS active drugs always have exclusive characteristics to penetrate into milk. Thus, if a drug is active in the central nervous system, to some extent higher milk levels can be expected. Opioids, and inhalational drugs they can simply enter milk.

- **Protein solubility**:
  The greater part of the drugs circulates in the maternal plasma bound to albumin. The UN bound part; remain freely soluble in the plasma. The un bound part of drugs transfer liberally into milk, while the bound parts stay in the maternal plasma unable to attain the tissues. Thus, drugs that have high maternal protein binding, more or less always produce lesser levels in milk.

**opioids chemical structure**:
- A basic amino group of different length
- An aromatic moiety
- A basophilic centre.

Those common features appear to be the essential structural for opioids (Casy 1971).

## Pharmacokinetic factors affect drug actions

Molecular weight.

Lipid solubility.

Protein binding.

Ionization.

## The effects are:

Increase or decrease the transport across membranes.

1-The receptor binding affinity.

2-The diffusion into the CNS.

3-The analgesic action.

## 5- Oral Bioavailability:

Oral Bioavailability is the amount of a drug that actually reaches the circulation of the individual

- are destroyed in the acidic milieu of the stomach,
  Others are rapidly extracted by the liver and fail to ever reach the infant's circulation.
- Some drugs are poorly absorbed when ingested with calcium rich foods and particularly milk.
- These absorption problems tend ultimately to reduce the overall effect of many drugs.

## 6- Molecular Weight:

- The lower the molecular weight of a drug, the more the penetrattion into human milk, because the diffusion throughout the alveolar epithelial cell is much easier.
- drugs with molecular weights less than 300 are considered smaller and will be likely to diffuse to milk in higher concentrations than those with higher molecular weights.

- With a molecular weight of 120, it rapidly equilibrates between the plasma and milk compartments
- Drugs with molecular weights of 600 or greater are improbable to diffuse into milk in high concentrations.

### 8- pKa:

The pKa of a drug is the pH at which the drug is equally ionic and nonionic. The more ionic a drug is, the less capable it is of transferring from the milk compartment to the maternal plasma compartment. Hence they become trapped in milk (ion-trapping). This term is useful, because drugs that have a pKa higher than 7.2 may be sequestered to a slightly higher degree than one with a lower pKa. Drugs with higher pKa generally have higher Milk:Plasma ratios. Hence, choose drugs with a lower pKa.

<u>**Opioids and breast lactation**</u> :


<u>**Fentanyl:**</u>

- Fentanyl, is lipophilic ,and crosses the blood-brain barrier rapidly in mutually directions. so, fentanyl acts rapidly ,and has a short duration of action .
- Fentanyl has high receptor affinity. Fentanyl binds tightly to a mu receptor; it may have a surprisingly long duration of action. The mu receptor dissociation constant for is 1.9.
- Elimination half-lives 3-7 hours for fentanyl.

- Fentanyl plasma protein binding capacity decreases with increasing ionization of the drug.

- Alterations in pH may affect its distribution between plasma and the central nervous system. It accumulates in skeletal muscle and fat, and is released slowly into the blood.

- Fentanyl, which is mainly transformed in the liver, demonstrates a high first pass clearance and releases approximately 75% of an intravenous dose in urine, mostly as metabolites with less than 10% representing the unchanged drug.

- About 9% of the dose is recovered in the feces, principally as metabolites.

- Plasma fentanyl levels of 0.2 to 1.2 mcg/L are required for analgesia via the nonepidural route and plasma levels over 1 to 2 mcg/L may cause respiratory depression. Plasma levels are markedly lower when the epidural route is used. The oral bioavailability of fentanyl is 33% in adults. The usual intravenous of fentanyl for an infant is 1 - 2 mcg/kg. Fentanyl is metabolized to norfentanyl and inactive metabolites.

- Fentanyl can increase serum prolactin. Nevertheless, prolactin level in a mother with established lactation has no effects.

- **Fentanyl when used in short procedures** epidurally or intravenously during labor or endoscopy fentanyl amount in breast milk is very small and are not detectable to affect breastfed infants. There is no need to discard milk before restart breastfeeding.] After general anesthesia, breastfeeding can be stared once the mother has recovered adequately to nurse her baby.

- Transdermal fentanyl in a dosage of 100 mcg/hour is invisible fentanyl concentrations in breast milk.

- In long procedures a combination of anesthetic agents is used, this can leads to decrease recovery of the mother or potentiate the effects fentayl.

- When mothers use oral fentanyl during breastfeeding  infants may has drowsiness, central nervous system depression and even death. Newborn infants appear to be mainly responsive to the effects of yet small dosages of fentanyl. It is best to provide pain control with a non narcotic analgesic, and control maternal intake of fentanyl to a few days at a minimal dosage in the company of close infant monitoring. If there is a sign of increased sleepiness difficulty breastfeeding, breathing difficulties, or flaccidity, call medical advice immediately.

**the effect of epidural fentanyl on breastfeeding initiation ,or duration are controversial, because of:**

Many different combinations of drugs.

Dosages and patient populations studied.

The variety of techniques used

Deficient design of many of the studies.

 Nevertheless, it appears that with good breastfeeding maintain, epidural fentanyl plus bupivacaine.

**Studies on the effect fentanyl on breast lactation (http://www.drugs.com/)**

(In 58 breastfeeding mothers who received an epidural fentanyl dosage greater than 150 mcg during labor, 21% reported more troubles in establishing breastfeeding at 24 hours after delivery compared to 10% of mothers who received to a lower dosage or to no fentanyl. There was no difference in breastfeeding difficulty noted between the groups 24 hours after delivery when the assessment was performed by a lactation consultant. Women in the high-dose group who could be contacted were more likely to discontinue breastfeeding by 6 weeks after delivery and there was a higher rate of breastfeeding discontinuation at 6 weeks among mothers who reported breastfeeding difficulty 24 hours after delivery.A relatively high dropout rate from the study at 6 weeks clouds the results.

A retrospective study of a random sample of 425 mothers delivering in a maternity unit found a dose-related increased risk of bottle feeding at hospital discharge associated with fentanyl administered during labor.

A prospective cohort study compared women who received continuous epidural analgesia with fentanyl and either bupivacaine or ropivacaine during labor and delivery (n = 52) to women who received no analgesia (n = 63). The average total fentanyl dosage was 124 mcg and the average total infusion time from start to delivery was 219 minutes. The study found no differences between the groups in breastfeeding effectiveness or infant neurobehavioral status at 8 to 12 hours postpartum or the number exclusively or partially breastfeeding at 4 weeks postpartum.

A randomized, prospective study measured infant breastfeeding behavior following epidural or intravenous fentanyl during delivery in 100 multiparous mothers undergoing cesarean section and delivering fullterm, healthy infants. Epidural fentanyl was given to 50 women in a dose of 100 to 150 mcg in divided doses followed by a continuous epidural infusion of 20 mcg/hour. Intravenous fentanyl was given to 50 women as a single dose of 50 mcg after delivery. Both groups received epidural or spinal bupivacaine in addition. A slight difference was seen in breastfeeding behavior between the groups, with the infants in the intravenous fentanyl group performing slightly worse than those in the epidural group. However, all mothers were able to breastfeed their infants at 24 hours. None had severe breastfeeding problems; 10 women in the epidural group reported mild or moderate problems and 7 women in the intravenous group reported breastfeeding problems.

Twenty mothers in the epidural group and 14 in the intravenous group used supplemental bottle feeding, with the difference not statistically significant.

A randomized, multicenter trial compared the initiation rate and duration of breastfeeding in women who received high-dose epidural bupivacaine alone, or one of two low-dose combinations of bupivacaine plus fentanyl. The average fentanyl dosages in the two groups were 97 and 151 mcg in the first stage of labor and 10 and 12 mcg of fentanyl during the second stage of labor, respectively, with great variability. A nonepidural matched control group was also compared. No differences in breastfeeding initiation rates or duration were found among the epidural and nonmedicated groups, but women in the nonepidural group who received systemic meperidine had a lower breastfeeding initiation rate than in the other groups.

A nonrandomized study in low-risk mother-infant pairs found that there was no difference overall in the amount of sucking by newborns, whether their mothers received bupivacaine plus fentanyl, or fentanyl alone by epidural infusion in various dosages, or received no analgesia for childbirth. In a subanalysis by sex and number of sucks, female infants were affected by high-dose bupivacaine and high-dose fentanyl, but male infant were not. However, the imbalances of many factors between the study groups make this study difficult to interpret.

In a prospective cohort study, 87 multiparous women who received epidural bupivacaine and fentanyl for pain control during labor and vaginal delivery. A loading dose of 0.125% bupivacaine with fentanyl 50-100 mcg. Epidural analgesia is maintained using 0.0625% bupivacaine and fentanyl 0.2 mcg/mL. The median dose of fentanyl received by the women was 151 mcg (range 30 to 570 mcg). The women completed questionnaires at 1 and 6 weeks postpartum regarding breastfeeding. Most women had prior experience with breastfeeding, support at home and ample time off from work. All women were breastfeeding at 1 week postpartum and 95.4% of women were breastfeeding at 6 weeks postpartum.

A nonrandomized study at one Italian hospital compared primaparous mothers undergoing vaginal delivery who received epidural analgesia (n = 64) to those who did not (n = 64). Mothers who requested the epidural analgesia received an initial dose of 100 mcg of fentanyl diluted to 10 mL with saline. After the initial fentanyl, doses of 15 to 20 mL of 0.1% ropivacaine were administered if needed. The only difference between the groups of mothers was a longer duration of labor among the treated mothers. The quality of infant nursing was equal between the 2 groups of infants on several measures; however, more infants in the treated group breastfed for less than 30 minutes at the first feeding.

A national survey of women and their infants from late pregnancy through 12 months postpartum compared the time of lactogenesis II in mothers who did and did not receive pain medication during labor. Categories of medication were spinal or epidural only, spinal or epidural plus another medication, and other pain medication only. Women who received medications from any of the categories had about twice the risk of having delayed lactogenesis II (>72 hours) compared to women who received no labor pain medication.

A randomized study compared the effects of cesarean section using general anesthesia, spinal anesthesia, or epidural anesthesia, to normal vaginal delivery on serum prolactin and oxytocin as well as time to initiation of lactation. General anesthesia was performed using propofol 2 mg/kg and rocuronium 0.6 mg/kg for induction, followed by sevoflurane and rocuronium 0.15 mg/kg as needed. After delivery, patients in all groups received an infusion of oxytocin 30 international units in 1 L of saline, and 0.2 mg of methylergonovine if they were not hypertensive. Fentanyl 1 to 1.5 mcg/kg was administered after delivery to the general anesthesia group. Patients in the general anesthesia group (n = 21) had higher post-procedure prolactin levels and a longer mean time to lactation initiation (25 hours) than in the other groups (10.8 to 11.8 hours). Postpartum oxytocin levels in the nonmedicated vaginal delivery group were higher than in the general and spinal anesthesia groups.

A randomized, nonblinded study compared the use of intramuscular meperidine 100 mg to intranasal (mean dose 486 mcg) or subcutaneous (mean dose 300 mcg) fentanyl for labor analgesia. More women in the meperidine group had difficulty establishing lactation (79%) than in the intranasal (39%) or subcutaneous (44%) fentanyl groups. Mothers who received meperidine reported more sedation, had longer labors, and their infants were).

## Morphine:

- Morphine is a long-acting opioid, its elimination half-lives 2-4 hours hours. It is eliminated more slowly from the body;

- its duration of action longer than fentanyl because it enters the central nervous system with difficulty due to cellular lipid barrier (blood-brain barrier).

- Its mu receptor binding affinities is similar to fentanyl (the mu receptor dissociation constant for is 2.0).

- it has minor e or no effect on breastfeeding


- more likely to be admitted to the nursery

### Remifentanil ( Ultiva):

- It is a potent ultra short-acting synthetic opioid.
- It is given to patients during surgery to relieve pain
- Remifentanil is used for sedation .
- It is used in general anesthesia.
- as well as combined with other medications for use in general anesthesia.
- The use of remifentanil has made possible the use of high-dose opioid and low-dose hypnotic anesthesia, due to synergism between remifentanil and different hypnotic drugs and volatile anesthetics.
- Most of other synthetic opioids are metabolized in the liver , remifentanil has an ester linkage which undergoes rapid hydrolysis by non-specific tissue, and plasma esterases. its context-sensitive half-life remains at 4 minutes after a 4 hour infusion .so the accumulation does not occur with remifentanil.
- Remifentanil is metabolized to a compound (remifentanil acid) which has 1/4600th the potency of the parent compound.
- Due to its quick metabolism, and the short effects remifentanil leasds to new possibilities in anesthesia.
- When remifentanil is used with a hypnotic (in induction of anesthesia it can be used in relative high doses. This is because remifentanil will be rapidly

- eliminated from the blood plasma on termination of the remifentanil infusion.
- Decreased doses of both remifentanil and hypnotics due to synergism between remifentanil and hypnotic drugs .
- Reduction of doses leads to more hemodynamic stability during surgery and decreases the post-operative recovery time.
- Theoretically it has less or no effect on breast feeding.
- The rapid recovery of mothers helps in rapid restoration of breast feeding.
- When used in vaginal delivery or cesarean section it leads to better Apgar score and less sedation of the baby make him take the earlier colostrums.
- There is no studies to assess the amount of Remifentanil after long duration infusion.

## Alfentanil:

- . Alfentanil is highly protein bound so it results in less transfer to breast milk than other opiates .

- When used epidurally or intravenously during labor or for a short time immediately postpartum, amounts of alfentanil in breast milk are small and with less or no adverse effects in breastfed infants.

- There are no published studies with repeated doses of intravenous alfentanil during established lactation.

- Caution is needed during using alfentanil especially in preterm babies.

- nonnarcotic analgesic and limit maternal intake of alfentanil.

- Careful monitoring. If the baby shows signs of increased sleepiness difficulty breastfeeding,

- Breathing difficulties or flaccidity a physician should be consulted immediately.

- Labor pain medication may delay the onset of lactation.

.

## Oxycodone

Oxycodone has an oral bioavailability of 60% to 87% in adults

- Oxycodone elimination is decreased in young infants, and much inter-individual variability exists.
- Oxycodone can be dangerous when used as an analgesic in newborns.
- Infant sedation is common, and well documented with maternal use of oxycodone.
- Newborns appear to be mainly sensitive to the effects of small dosages of Oxycodone.
- It is best to limit maternal intake of oral oxycodone (and combinations) to a few days.
- A maximum oxycodone dosage of 30 mg daily is suggested.
- Oxycodone elimination is decreased in young infants with much inter-individual variability.

- Monitor the infant closely for drowsiness, adequate weight gain, and developmental milestones, especially in younger, exclusively breastfed infants.

- If the baby shows signs of increased sleepiness (more than usual), difficulty breastfeeding, breathing difficulties, or flaccidity, a physician should be consulted immediately.

- Other agents are preferred over oxycodone during breastfeeding.


## Hydromorphone :

- Limited data indicate that hydromorphone is excreted into breastmilk in small amounts. Maternal use of oral narcotics during breastfeeding can cause infant drowsiness, central nervous system depression and even death.

- In adults, hydromorphone has an oral bioavailability of 62% and is metabolized to inactive metabolites. While not commonly used in infants, an appropriate dose for this age group is 10 mcg/kg parenterally or 30 mcg/kg orally every 4 hours as needed.

- Newborn infants seem to be particularly sensitive to the effects of even small dosages of narcotic analgesics.

- Once the mother's milk comes in, it is best to provide pain control with a nonnarcotic analgesic and limit maternal intake of hydromorphone to a few days at a low dosage with close infant monitoring.

- If the baby shows signs of increased sleepiness (more than usual), difficulty breastfeeding, breathing difficulties, or limpness, a physician should be contacted immediately.

  Eight lactating women (time postpartum not given) were given a single 2 mg intranasal dose of hydromorphone. Milk was collected 7 times, beginning 2 hours after and ending 24 hours after the dose. Peak milk levels occurred 2 hours after the dose. The half-life of elimination from milk was 10.5 hours. The reported average milk level, over the 24 hour period after the single dose, was about 1 mcg/L. The authors calculated that an exclusively breastfed infant would receive 0.67% of the maternal weight-adjusted dosage. Using the average milk level reported in this study, an exclusively breastfed infant would receive 0.15 mcg/kg daily from a single maternal 2 mg intranasal hydromorphone dose.

- Narcotics can increase serum prolactin. However, the prolactin level in a mother with established lactation may not affect her ability to breastfeed.

## Butorphanol :

- Limited data indicate that butorphanol is excreted into breastmilk in small amounts. Butorphanol is poorly orally absorbed,

- so it is unlikely to adversely affect the breastfed infant.

- In adults, the oral bioavailability of butorphanol is 17% while the intranasal bioavailability is 70%. Butorphanol is metabolized to inactive metabolites. Intranasal and parenteral doses of 25 to 30 mcg/kg have been used in infants as young as 6 months for postoperative analgesia.

- Narcotics and narcotic agonist-antagonists can increase serum prolactin .However; the prolactin level in a mother with established lactation may not affect her ability to breastfeed.

- There is no published experience with repeated, high, intravenous or intranasal doses of butorphanol during breastfeeding should be avoided.

- Other agents may be preferred in these situations, especially while nursing a newborn or preterm infant.

- Monitor the infant for drowsiness, adequate weight gain, and developmental milestones, especially in younger, exclusively breastfed infants.

- As with other narcotics, once the mother's milk comes in, it is best to limit maternal intake and to supplement analgesia with a nonnarcotic analgesic, if necessary for pain control. If the baby shows signs of increased sleepiness (more than usual), difficulty breastfeeding, breathing difficulties, or limpness, a physician should be contacted immediately. Labor pain medication may delay the onset of lactation.

- Twelve lactating women were given a single butorphanol dose at 2 to 4 days postpartum. Six of these women were given a 2 mg single intramuscular dose and 6 others were given a single 8 mg oral dose. Milk was sampled 3 times after the dose. The reported average milk levels were 1.5, 0.7 and 0.3 mcg/L at 2, 4 and 8 hours, respectively, after the 2 mg intramuscular dose. The average milk levels after the 8 mg oral dose were 3.6, 1.8 and 1 mcg/L at 3, 5 and 8 hours, respectively. The half-life of elimination from milk was about 2 hours. Using the data from this study, doses of butorphanol 2 mg intramuscularly or 8 mg orally will result in average milk levels of 0.7 and 2 mcg/L, respectively, over 8 hours after the dose. Using these calculated average milk levels, an exclusively breastfed infant would receive 0.035 mcg/kg from a 2 mg intramuscular maternal dose of butorphanol, and 0.1 mcg/kg from an 8 mg oral maternal dose of butorphanol,

- from milk ingested up through 8 hours after the dose. These amounts represent 0.11% and 0.08% of the maternal weight-adjusted dosages, respectively.

- A study compared women who received butorphanol or nalbuphine during labor (n = 26) to those who received no analgesia (n = 22). The time to effective breastfeeding was longer (46.5 minutes) in the analgesia group than in the no analgesia group (35.4 minutes)

- A national survey of women and their infants from late pregnancy through 12 months postpartum compared the time of lactogenesis II in mothers who did and did not receive pain medication during labor. Categories of medication were spinal or epidural only, spinal or epidural plus another medication, and other pain medication only. Women who received medications from any of the categories had about twice the risk of having delayed lactogenesis II (>72 hours) compared to women who received no labor pain medication..

## Hypnotics ,and breast lactation:

## Na Thiopental:

- Small amounts of thiopental may appear in the milk of nursing mothers following administration of large doses.

- The manufacturer makes no recommendation regarding the use of thiopental during lactation.

- A normal dose of sodium thiopental (usually 4–6 mg/kg) given to a pregnant woman for rapid sequence induction for cesarean section it rapidly makes her unconscious, but the baby remains conscious.

- Large or repeated doses can depress the baby.

- Thiopental rapidly and easily crosses the blood brain barrier as it is a highly lipophilic molecule. The short duration of action of sodium thiopental is due almost completely to its redistribution away from central circulation towards muscle and fat tissue,

- Due to its very high fat: water partition coefficient (aprx 10), leading to sequestration in fat tissue. Once redistributed, the free fraction in the blood is metabolized in the liver.

- Sodium thiopental is mainly metabolized to <u>pentobarbital</u>, 5-ethyl-5-(1'-methyl-3'-hydroxybutyl)-2-thiobarbituric acid, and 5-ethyl-5-(1'-methyl-3'-carboxypropyl)-2-thiobarbituric acid.

**Midazolam**

- A short-acting hypnotic-sedative drug with anxiolytic and amnestic properties. It is used in dentistry, cardiac surgery, endoscopic procedures, as preanesthetic medication, and as an adjunct to local anesthesia.
- The short duration and cardiorespiratory stability makes it useful in poor-risk, elderly, and cardiac patients. It is water-soluble at pH less than 4 and lipid-soluble at physiological pH
- Benzodiazepine pharmacologic effects appear to result from reversible interactions with the (gamma)-amino butyric acid (GABA) benzodiazepine receptor in the CNS, the major inhibitory neurotransmitter in the central nervous system. The action of midazolam is readily reversed by the benzodiazepine receptor antagonist, flumazenil.

- Benzodiazepine pharmacologic effects appear to result from reversible interactions with the (gamma)-amino butyric acid (GABA) benzodiazepine receptor in the CNS, the major inhibitory neurotransmitter in the central nervous system. The action of midazolam is readily reversed by the benzodiazepine receptor antagonist, flumazenil.

- Midazolam is primarily metabolized in the liver and gut by human cytochrome P450 IIIA4 (CYP3A4) to its pharmacologic active metabolite, α-hydroxymidazolam, followed by glucuronidation of the α–hydroxyl metabolite which is present in unconjugated and conjugated forms in human plasma. The α- hydroxymidazolam glucuronide is then excreted in urine. No significant amount of parent drug or metabolites is extractable from urine before beta-glucuronidase and sulfatase deconjugation, indicating that the urinary metabolites are excreted mainly as conjugates. The amount of midazolam excreted unchanged in the urine when given intravenously is less than 0.5%. 45% to 57% of the dose was excreted in the urine as 1-hydroxymethyl midazolam conjugate.

- It is excreted into human milk in very small amounts.

- Sedation is a theoretic concern but has not been reported.

- Midazolam is described by the American Academy of Pediatrics as a drug "whose effect on nursing infants is unknown but may be of concern"

## Propofol:

- Propofol is highly protein-bound *in vivo* and is metabolised by <u>conjugation</u> in the liver.

- The <u>half-life of elimination</u> of propofol was estimated to be between 2 and 24 hours.

- propofol is rapidly distributed into peripheral tissues so its duration of clinical effect is much shorter.

- A single dose of propofol typically wears off within minutes.

- Propofol can be given for short or prolonged sedation, as well as for general anesthesia.

- Its use is not associated with nausea as is often seen with opioid medications.

- The amount of propofol received by the infant during breast-feeding is very small and is not absorbed by the infant.

- Many clinicians feel breast-feeding is safe for the infant after maternal administration of propofol. One group of women undergoing Cesarean section was given a mean dose of 2.55 mg/kg. Another group was given 2.51 mg/kg plus a mean infusion of 5.08 mg/kg/hour. Breast milk/colostrum samples were collected between 4 and 24 hours after delivery. Propofol concentrations varied between 0.048 mcg/mL and 0.74 mcg/mL.

- The highest levels occurred 4 to 5 hours after delivery.

- One small study has reported the pharmacokinetic data of five lactating women who underwent induction of anesthesia with propofol. In 24 hours of milk collection, an average of 0.027% (0.004% to 0.082%) of the maternal propofol was collected in the milk representing an average of 0.025% of the elimination clearance of the drug. The author of the study concluded that the amount of propofol excreted into the milk within 24 hours of induction of anesthesia provided insufficient justification to interrupt breast-feeding.

- Propofol is excreted into human milk. The manufacturer recommends that propofol not be used during nursing because the effects of oral absorption of propofol in the infant are unknown.

- Amounts of propofol in milk are very small and are not expected to be absorbed by the infant.

- Some studies recommend stop nursing for an indefinite time after propofol administration .Most of the studies recommended   that breastfeeding can be resumed once the mother has recovered sufficiently from general anesthesia to nurse, and that removal milk is avoidable.

- General anesthesia for cesarean section using propofol as an  induction drug may delay the onset of  lactation.

- In one case, milk was noted to be green in color 8 hours after a procedure in which propofol was administered; however, several other medications were also used during the procedure.

## Etomidate:

- Amounts of etomidate in milk are very small, and decrease rapidly.

- Etomidate is rapidly metabolized by hydrolysis of the ethyl ester side chain to its carboxylic acid ester, resulting in a water-soluble, pharmacologically inactive compound.

- Hepatic microsomal enzymes and plasma esterase are responsible for this hydrolysis. Hydrolysis is nearly complete, as evidenced by recovery of < 3% of an administered dose of etomidate metabolism as unchanged drug in urine. Seventy six per cent is bound to plasma protein mainly albumin.

- Accessible data show that no waiting period is needed before resuming breastfeeding after etomidate anesthesia.

- Twenty women undergoing cesarean section received 0.3 mg/kg of etomidate intravenously for induction of anesthesia. Average colostrum levels were 79.3 mcg/L (range 0 to 420 mcg/L) at 30 minutes and 16.2 mcg/L (range 0 to 60 mcg/L) at 2 hours after the dose. Etomidate was not detected in any colostrum samples 4 hours after the dose

- Breastfeeding can be resumed as soon as the mother has recovered sufficiently from general anesthesia to nurse.

- When a combination of anesthetic agents is used for a procedure, recommendations for the most problematic medication used during the procedure must be followed.

## Methohexital :

- Metabolism of methohexital is primarily hepatic (i.e., taking place in the liver) via demethylation and oxidation.

- Side-chain oxidation is the primary means of metabolism involved in the termination of the drug's biological activity.

- Protein binding is approximately 73% for methohexital.

- Amounts of methohexital in milk are very small.

- Existing data indicate that no waiting period is required before resuming breastfeeding after a single dose of methohexital.

- Breastfeeding can be resumed as soon as the mother has recovered sufficiently to nurse.

- When a combination of anesthetic agents is used for a procedure, follow the recommendations for the most problematic medication used during the procedure.

- Nine women who were at least 1 month postpartum received between 120 and 150 mg of methohexital intravenously for induction of general anesthesia for bilateral tubal ligation. Milk samples were obtained in the recovery room after surgery, the evening of surgery and on the day after surgery. The highest milk level was found at 63 minutes after the dose in one woman. Milk levels 1 to 2 hours after the dose ranged from 100 to 407 mcg/L (n = 5); levels 2 to 4 hours after the dose ranged from 39 to 199 mcg/L (n = 4); levels 8 to 10 hours after the dose ranged from undetectable (<20 mcg/L) to 65 mcg/L (n = 9). Methohexital was not detectable in the breast milk of any woman 24 to 48 hours after the dose. The authors estimated that the typical breastfed infant would receive a maximum single dose of 0.04 mg of methohexital in a 100 mL feeding 1 hour after the dose or between 0.1 to 0.8% of the maternal weight-adjusted dosage.

## Inhalational anesthetics and breast feeding:

## Sevoflurane:

- Sevoflurane, USP, a volatile liquid for inhalation, a nonflammable and nonexplosive liquid administered by vaporization, is a halogenated general inhalation anesthetic drug. Sevoflurane is fluoromethyl 2,2,2-trifluoro-1-(trifluoromethyl) ethyl ether, ($C_4H_3F_7O$),

- Sevoflurane alkaline degradation occurs by two pathways.

- The first results from the loss of hydrogen fluoride with the formation of pentafluoroisopropenyl fluoromethyl ether (PIFE, $C_4H_2F_6O$), also known as Compound A, and trace amounts of pentafluoromethoxy isopropyl fluoromethyl ether, (PMFE, $C_5H_6F_6O$), also known as Compound B.

- The second pathway for degradation of Sevoflurane which occurs primarily in the presence of desiccated $CO_2$ absorbents, is discussed later.

- In the first pathway, the defluorination pathway, the production of degradants in the anesthesia circuit results from the extraction of the acidic proton in the presence of a strong base (KOH and/or NaOH) forming an alkene (Compound A) from Sevoflurane similar to formation of 2-bromo-2-chloro-1,1-difluoro ethylene (BCDFE) from halothane. Laboratory simulations have shown that the concentration of these degradants is inversely correlated with the fresh gas flow rate.

Caution is recommended. Excreted into human milk: Unknown Excreted into animal milk: Data not available Comments: -Advice women to skip breastfeeding for 48 hours after administration and discard milk produced during this period.

## Desflurane :

- Desflurane (1,2,2,2-tetrafluoroethyl difluoromethyl ether) is a highly fluorinated methyl ethyl ether used for maintenance of general anesthesia.

- There is no published experience with desflurane during breastfeeding.

- The serum half-life of desflurane in the mother is short , The serum half-life of desflurane is less than 3 minutes, and the drug is not expected to be absorbed by the infant,

- There is need for waiting period or discarding of milk.

- Breastfeeding can be resumed as soon as the mother has recovered sufficiently from general anesthesia to nurse.

- When a combinations of anesthetic agents ,and narcotics are used for a procedure, recommendations for the most problematic medication used during the procedure must be followed..

,

## Non steroidal drugs ,and breast lactation:

## Acetaminophen

- Acetaminophen is a good choice for analgesia, and fever reduction in nursing mothers.

- Amounts in milk are much less than doses usually given to infants. Adverse effects in breastfed infants appear to be rare.

- A single oral dose of 650 mg of acetaminophen was given to 12 nursing mothers who were 2 to 22 months postpartum. Peak milk levels of 10 to 15 mg/L occurred between 1 and 2 hours after the dose in all patients. Acetaminophen was undetectable (<0.5 mg/L) in all mothers 12 hours after the dose. The authors calculated that an infant who ingested 90 mL of breastmilk every 3 hours would receive an average of 0.88 mg of acetaminophen or 0.14% (range 0.04 to 0.23%) of the mother's absolute dosage.Using data from this study, an infant would receive a maximum of about 2% of the maternal weight-adjusted dosage.

- Three women took a single 500 mg dose of acetaminophen. Peak milk levels averaging 4.2 mg/L occurred within 2 hours after the dose. Using data from this study, an infant would receive a maximum of about 3.6% of the maternal weight-adjusted dosage.

- Four women who were 2 to 8 months postpartum were given a single 1 gram dose of acetaminophen. Peak milk levels occurred between 1 and 2.5 hours after the dose. The authors estimated that a breastfed infant would receive an average of 1.1% and a maximum of 1.8% of the maternal weight-adjusted dosage. This dose is about 0.5% of the lowest recommended infant dose of acetaminophen.

- . No acetaminophen was detected in the urine of 12 breastfed infants aged 2 to 22 months after maternal ingestion of 650 mg of acetaminophen.

- Urine was collected for 1 to 3.5 hours after nursing in 6 infants aged 2 to 6 days whose mothers received 1 to 2 grams of acetaminophen 2 to 4 hours before nursing their infant. Infants excreted an average of 401 mcg of acetaminophen and its metabolites in urine during the collection interval. These neonates excreted a greater percentage of drug as acetaminophen and much less as the sulfate metabolite than adults.

- A maculopapular rash on the upper trunk and face of a 2-month-old infant was probably caused by acetaminophen in breastmilk. The rash occurred after 2 days of therapy in the mother at a dose of 1 gram at bedtime. It subsided when the drug was discontinued and recurred 2 weeks later after another acetaminophen dose of 1 gram was taken by the mother.

- Two papers report 14 women who breastfed after taking acetaminophen or its prodrug phenacetin with no adverse effects to their infants.In a telephone follow-up study, mothers reported no side effects among 43 infants exposed to acetaminophen in breastmilk.

- Two clinicians speculated that breastmilk exposure to acetaminophen during breastfeeding might be a risk factor for asthma and wheezing in the breastfed infants based on their personal observations. However, these observations were uncontrolled and cannot be considered to be valid proof of an association.

## Ibuprofen

- It is extremely low levels in breast milk

- Short half-life and use in infants in doses much higher than those excreted in breast milk, ibuprofen is a preferred choice as an analgesic or anti inflammatory agent in nursing mothers.Two early studies attempted measurement of ibuprofen in milk. In one, the patient's dose was 400 mg twice daily, while in the second study of 12 patients, the dose was 400 mg every 6 h

- Ibuprofen was undetectable in breastmilk in both studies (<0.5 and 1 mg/L, respectively).

- A later study using a more sensitive assay found ibuprofen in the breastmilk of one woman who took 6 doses of 400 mg orally over a 42.5 hours. A milk ibuprofen level of 13 mcg/L was detected 30 minutes after the first dose. The highest level measured was 180 mcg/L about 4 hours after the third dose, 20.5 hours after the first dose. The authors estimated that the infant would receive about 17 mcg/kg daily (100 mcg daily) with the maternal dose of approximately 1.2 grams daily. This dose represents 0.0008% of the maternal weight-adjusted dosage[3] and 0.06% of the commonly accepted infant dose of 30 mg/kg daily (10 mg/kg every 8 hours).

- Single milk samples were taken from 13 women between 1.5 and 8 hours after the third dose of ibuprofen in a daily dosage regimen averaging 1046 mg daily (range 400 to 1200 mg daily). The mean milk concentration was 361 mcg/L (range 164 to 590 mcg/L). The mean weight-adjusted percentage of the maternal dosage (relative infant dosage [RID]) was estimated to be <0.38%; however, the RID varied with the time postpartum and the milk protein content. The RID was highest in the colostral phase when the milk protein content was the highest (RID 0.6%). The estimated mean dosage for a fully breastfed infants was 68 mcg/kg daily.

- At least 23 cases are reported in the literature in which infants (ages not stated) were breastfed during maternal ibuprofen use with no adverse effects reported.

## Flurbiprofen :

- Because of the low levels of flurbiprofen in breastmilk and its short half-life it is unlikely to adversely affect the breastfed infant, especially if the infant is older than 2 months

- Ten women who were at least 1 month postpartum were given a single 100 mg tablet of flurbiprofen. Flurbiprofen was undetectable (<70 mcg/L) in the milk of 5 of the women. In the remaining 5 women, an average peak milk level of 92 mcg/L occurred at about 3 hours after the dose. Flurbiprofen was undetectable in any mother's milk by 24 hours after the dose.[1] Using data from this study, a fully breastfed infant would ingest an estimated maximum of 2.2 mcg/kg/day after this maternal dosage or about 0.1% of the maternal weight-adjusted dosage.

- Twelve women who were 3 to 5 days postpartum received flurbiprofen 50 mg orally four times a day for 9 doses over 3 days. Milk samples were collected at various unspecified times during this regimen. Flurbiprofen was undetectable (<50 mcg/L) in all but 3 milk samples.

- One woman had levels of 70 mcg/L 1 hour after her first dose and 60 mcg/L just before her second dose. Another woman had a milk flurbiprofen concentration of 80 mcg/L 2 hours after her last dose. The authors estimated that the maximum dose that a completely breastfed infant would ingest is less than 0.5% of the maternal weight-adjusted dosage.

**Naproxen**:

- Limited information indicates that levels of naproxen in breastmilk are low and adverse effects in breastfed infants are apparently uncommon.

- However, because of naproxen's long half-life and reported serious adverse reaction in a breastfed neonate, other agents may be preferred while nursing a newborn or preterm infant.

- *Maternal Levels.* Peak milk naproxen levels in a 5-month postpartum patient were 1.1 to 1.3 mg/L while taking oral naproxen 250 mg twice daily and 2.4 mg/L with a dose of 375 mg twice daily. Peak milk levels occurred 4 to 5 hours after the dose and fell slowly over 12 to 24 hours. From urinary excretion data the authors estimated that the infant received 0.26% of the mother's total dose or 1.9% of the maternal weight-adjusted dosage.

- Using the peak milk level data, the estimated maximum intake of an exclusively breastfed infant would be 2.2 to 2.8% of the maternal weight-adjusted dosage, not including the contribution of any glucuronide metabolite.

- Naproxen possibly caused prolonged bleeding time, thrombocytopenia and acute anemia in one 7-day-old infant in a mother also taking bacampicillin.

- In one telephone follow-up study of 20 infants exposed to naproxen during breastfeeding, 2 mothers reported drowsiness and 1 reported vomiting in their infants. None of the reactions required medical attention.

- A randomized study compared naproxen and tramadol for post-cesarean section pain. Patients received the drugs either on a fixed schedule or as needed. No difference in breastfeeding rates were seen among the groups.

## Piroxicam

- Low amounts of piroxicam in milk and failure to detect piroxicam or its metabolites in the urine of 2 older infants indicates that it would not be expected to cause adverse effects in older breastfed infants.

- Because there is no published experience with piroxicam during breastfeeding in the newborn period, shorter-acting agents may be preferred while nursing a newborn or preterm infant.

- Peak milk levels of 170 and 220 mcg/L were found in the milk of 2 women who were taking piroxicam 20 and 40 mg daily, respectively. The time of the peak milk levels were 12 and 4 hours after the dose, respectively, in the 2 women.

- Maximum milk piroxicam levels averaging 40 mcg/L were found in 3 women during the first week of therapy with oral piroxicam 20 mg daily. After steady-state was attained in these 3 women plus one additional woman, milk levels averaged 102 mcg/L during the first 12 hours after the dose and 73 mcg/L during the period of 13 to 24 hours after the dose. A nursing infant would receive an estimated average 3.5% and maximum 6.3% of the weight-adjusted maternal dosage.

- . No piroxicam could be detected in the serum of an 13-month-old infant whose mother had been taking 20 mg daily of piroxicam for 4 months.[1]

- Neither piroxicam nor its conjugates could be detected (<15 mcg/L) in the urine of one infant after 52 days of maternal therapy with 20 mg daily.

- No adverse effects were found in the breastfed infant of a patient receiving 20 mg of piroxicam daily for 4 months starting the 9th month postpartum.

- Four infants 3 to 4.5 months of age remained healthy during long-term therapy of their mothers with piroxicam 20 mg daily.

### Indomethacin:

- Because of the low levels of indomethcin in breastmilk and therapeutic administration directly to infants, it is acceptable to use in nursing mothers.

- However, other agents with more published information on use during lactation may be preferable, especially while nursing a newborn or preterm infant.

- In one study, 15 women who were less than 1 week postpartum took indomethacin in dosages ranging from 75 mg orally to 300 mg rectally daily (0.94 to 4.29 mg/kg daily). Milk samples were taken before and after feeding at times ranging from 0.7 to 21.4 hours after the last dose. In 11 of the women, indomethacin was undetectable (<20 mcg/L) in milk. Assuming that undetectable milk levels had the concentration of the assay limit, the average dosage excreted in milk was 0.27% of maternal weight-adjusted dosage.

- However, the excretion of the glucuronide metabolite into milk was not measured and it could be absorbed as indomethacin by a newborn.

- Eight women donated milk on days 4, 12 and 26 postpartum for an in vitro measurement of protein binding and lipid partitioning of indomethacin in milk. Results were used to estimate passage into milk using physicochemical principles. The authors calculated that a breastfed infant would receive about 0.5% of the maternal weight-adjusted dosage or about 3% of the neonatal dose used to treat patent ductus arteriosus with a maternal dosage of 75 mg daily. This study did not account for possible contribution to the infant's dosage by the glucuronide metabolite.

- In 6 of 7 infants breastfed during maternal indomethacin use of 75 mg orally to 300 mg rectally daily, the drug was undetectable (<20 mcg/L) in plasma. One infant had a plasma level of 47 mcg/L at 1.2 hours after the midpoint of the breastfeed. This infant's mother was taking 2.94 mg/kg daily of indomethacin and had a milk indomethacin level of 111 mcg/L 2.3 hours after the dose.

- In one case report, a breastfeeding mother had been taking daily doses of indomethacin that increased to 200 mg (3 mg/kg) from the fourth to the sixth day postpartum. On the same day that indomethacin was stopped, the infant had a generalized seizure, followed by another on the next day. No metabolic findings could account for the convulsions and no indomethacin levels were measured in the mother or infant. This case was rated as indomethacin possibly causing the seizure; however later studies and the established therapeutic use of indomethacin in newborns make this causality seem unlikely.

- In one study, 7 women breastfed their neonates while taking indomethacin. No adverse effects were noted in any of the infants.

## Tips for post operative analgesia:

Avoid drug therapy when possible

1-Use regional analgesia when possible.

2-Medications that are safe for use directly in an infant of the nursing infant's age are generally safe for the breast-feeding mother.

3-drugs that are safe in pregnancy are not always safe in breast-feeding mothers.

4-you can use consistent references for getting information on medications in breast milk.

5-the lowest effective maternal dose should be given. Moreover, infant exposure can be further reduced if breast-feeding is avoided at times of peak drug concentration in milk.

6- Follow up the infant while continues breast-feeding for possible adverse effects.

7-Breast-feeding during maternal treatment with paracetamol (acetaminophen) should be regarded as being safe.

8-Short term use of nonsteroidal anti-inflammatory drugs appears to be well-suited with breast-feeding.

9-For long term treatment, short-acting agents without active metabolites, such as ibuprofen, should possibly be preferred.


10-The use of aspirin (acetylsalicylic acid) in single doses should not pose any significant risks to the suckling infant.

11-Use of codeine is may be compatible with breast-feeding, although the effects of long term exposure have not been fully studied.

12-For propoxyphene, it seems unlikely that the suckling infant will ingest amounts that will cause any detrimental effects during short term treatment. However, it cannot be excluded that significant amounts of the metabolite norpropoxyphene may arise in the suckling infant during long term exposure.

13-Treatment of the mother with single doses of morphine or pethidine (meperidine) is not expected to cause any risk for the suckling infant.

14-Repeated administration of pethidine, in contrast to morphine, affects the suckling infant negatively. Thus, morphine should be preferred in lactating mothers.

15- However, during long term treatment with morphine, the importance of uninterrupted breast-feeding should be assessed on an individual basis against the potential risk of adverse drug effects in the infant.

# References:

1. Vargo JJ, Delegge MH, Feld AD et al. Multisociety sedation curriculum for gastrointestinal endoscopy. Gastroenterology. 2012;143:e18-41

2. Dailland P, Cockshott ID, Didier Lirzin J et al. Intravenous propofol during cesarean section: placental transfer, concentrations in breast milk, and neonatal effects. A preliminary study. Anesthesiology. 1989;71:827-34.

3. Nitsun M, Szokol JW, Saleh HJ, Murphy GS, Vender JS, Luong L et al. Pharmacokinetics of midazolam, propofol, and fentanyl transfer to human breast milk. Clin Pharmacol Ther. 2006;79:549-57

4. Shergill AK, Ben-Menachem T, Chandrasekhara V et al. Guidelines for endoscopy in pregnant and lactating women. Gastrointest Endosc. 2012;76:18-24.

5. Schmitt JP, Schwoerer D, Diemunsch P et al. [Passage of propofol in the colostrum. Preliminary data]. Ann Fr Anesth Reanim. 1987;6:267-8.

6. Birkholz T, Eckardt G, Renner S et al. Green breast milk after propofol administration. Anesthesiology. 2009;111:1168-9

7. Stuttmann R , Schafer C, Hilbert P et al. The breast feeding mother and xenon anaesthesia: four case reports. Breast feeding and xenon anaesthesia. BMC Anesthesiol. 2010;10:1.

8. Kutlucan L, Seker IS, Demiraran Y et al. Effects of different anesthesia protocols on lactation in the postpartum period. J Turkish German Gynecol Assoc Artemis. 2014;15:233-8.

9.Veselis RA, Reinsel RA, Feshchenko VA, Wroński M (October 1997). "The comparative amnestic effects of midazolam, propofol, thiopental, and fentanyl at equisedative concentrations". *Anesthesiology* **87** (4): 749–64

10. Shergill AK, Ben-Menachem T, Chandrasekhara V et al. Guidelines for endoscopy in pregnant and lactating women. Gastrointest Endosc. 2012;76:18-24.

11. Vargo JJ, Delegge MH, Feld AD et al. Multisociety sedation curriculum for gastrointestinal endoscopy. Gastroenterology. 2012;143:e18-41

12. Reynolds F. Labour analgesia and the baby: good news is no news. Int J Obstet Anesth. 2011;20:38-504.

13. Loubert C, Hinova A, Fernando R. Update on modern neuraxial analgesia in labour: a review of the literature of the last 5 years. Anaesthesia. 2011;66:191-212.

14. Shrestha B, Devgan A, Sharma M. Effects of maternal epidural analgesia on the neonate - a prospective cohort study. Ital J Pediatr. 2014;40:99.

15. Zuppa A, Alighieri G, Riccardi R et al. Epidural analgesia, neonatal care and breastfeeding. Ital J Pediatr. 2014;40: 82.

16. Madej TH, Strunin L. Comparison of epidural fentanyl with sufentanil. Anaesthesia. 1987;42:1156-61

17. Steer PL, Biddle CJ, Marley WS et al. Concentration of fentanyl in colostrum after an analgesic dose. Can J Anaesth. 1992;39:231-5.

18. Leuschen MP, Wolf LJ, Rayburn WF. Fentanyl excretion in breast milk. Clin Pharm. 1990;9:336-7.

19. Nitsun M, Szokol JW L et al. Pharmacokinetics of midazolam, propofol, and fentanyl transfer to human breast milk. Clin Pharmacol Ther. 2006;79:549-57.

20. Goma HM, Said RN, El-Ela AM. Study of the newborn feeding behaviors and fentanyl concentration in colostrum after an analgesic dose of epidural and intravenous fentanyl in cesarean section. Saudi Med J. 2008;29:678-82.

21. Cohen RS. Fentanyl transdermal analgesia during pregnancy and lactation. J Hum Lact. 2009;25:359-61

22. Ekwa-Ekoko C, Beilin Y, Abramowitz S, Holzman I , Weiser J, Kavanaugh N. Labor epidural fentanyl and new-born breast-feeding. Pediatr Res. 2000;47 (4 Pt 2):187A.

23. Beilin Y, Bodian CA, Weiser J et al. Effect of labor epidural analgesia with and without fentanyl on infant breast-feeding: a prospective, randomized, double-blind study. Anesthesiology. 2005;103:1211-7

24. Halpern SH, Ioscovich A. Epidural analgesia and breast-feeding. Anesthesiology. 2005;103:1111-2.

25. Frecska E, Perenyi A, Arato M. Blunted prolactin response to fentanyl in depression. Normalizing effect of partial sleep deprivation. Psychiatry Res. 2003;118:155-64.

26. Naito Y, Tamai S, Fukata J et al. Comparison of endocrinological stress response associated with transvaginal ultrasound-guided oocyte pick-up under halothane anaesthesia and neuroleptanaesthesia. Can J Anaesth. 1989;36:633-6.

27. Jordan S, Emery S, Bradshaw C et al. The impact of intrapartum analgesia on infant feeding . BJOG. 2005;112:927-34

28. Chang ZM, Heaman MI. Epidural analgesia during labor and delivery: effects on the initiation and continuation of effective breastfeeding. J Hum Lact. 2005;21:305-14

29. Wilson MJ, Macarthur C, Cooper GM et al. Epidural analgesia and breastfeeding: a randomised controlled trial of epidural techniques with and without fentanyl and a non-epidural comparison group. Anaesthesia. 2009.

30. Bell AF, White-Traut R, Medoff-Cooper B. Neonatal neurobehavioral organization after exposure to maternal epidural analgesia in labor. J Obstet Gynecol Neonatal Nurs. 2010;39:178-90.

31. Wieczorek PM, Guest S, Balki M et al. Breastfeeding success rate after vaginal delivery can be high despite the use of epidural fentanyl: an observational cohort study. Int J Obstet Anesth. 2010;19:273-7

32. Gizzo S, Di Gangi S, Saccardi C et al. Epidural analgesia during labor: impact on delivery outcome, neonatal well-being, and early breastfeeding. Breastfeed Med. 2012;7:262-8

33. Lind JN, Perrine CG, Li R. Relationship between use of labor pain medications and delayed onset of lactation. J Hum Lact. 2014;30:167-73.

34. Kutlucan L, Seker IS, Demiraran Y et al. Effects of different anesthesia protocols on lactation in the postpartum period. J Turkish German Gynecol Assoc Artemis. 2014;15:233-8.

35. Fleet J, Belan I, Jones M et al. A comparison of fentanyl with pethidine for pain relief during childbirth: A randomised controlled trial. BJOG. 2015.

36."WHO Model List of Essential Medicines" (PDF). World Health Organization. March 2005. Retrieved 2006-03-12.

37."Death Penalty Opposition: EU Set to Ban Export of Drug Used in US Executions". Spiegel Online International. Retrieved 23 January 2014.

38. Morgan, DJ; Blackman, GL; Paull, JD; Wolf, LJ (1981). "Pharmacokinetics and plasma binding of thiopental. II: Studies at cesarean section". *Anesthesiology* **54** (6): 474–80.

**39**. http://www.trauma.org/archive/anaesthesia/barbcoma.html

**40**.Pérez-Bárcena J; Barceló B; Homar J et al. (February 2005). "[Comparison of the effectiveness of pentobarbital and thiopental in patients with refractory intracranial hypertension. Preliminary report of 20 patients]". *Neurocirugia (Astur)* (in Spanish) **16**(1): 5–12; discussion 12–3. PMID 15756405. Retrieved 2008-07-18.

**41**. Krishnamurthy, KB; Drislane FW. "Depth of EEG suppression and outcome in barbiturate anesthetic treatment for refractory status epilepticus". *Epilepsia*. 1999 Jun; **40** (6): 759–762.

*42.* Royal Dutch Society for the Advancement of Pharmacy (1994). "Administration and Compounding of Euthanasic Agents". The Hague. Retrieved 2008-07-18.

**43**. "Ohio executes inmate with 1-drug lethal injection". Associated Press. December 2001. Retrieved 2009-12-08.

**44**. Martinez, Edecio (8 December 2009). "Kenneth Biros Execution: Ohio Man First to Die Under 1-Drug Thiopental Sodium Method". *CBS News*.

**45**.Sullivan, Jennifer (10 September 2010). "Killer on death row 16-1/2 years is executed".*The Seattle Times*

46. BC: US lethal injection drug faces UK export restrictions, 29 November 2010

47. UK government Web site: Controls on Torture Goods

48.EU Council Regulation (EU) No 1352/2011

49."Truth serum used on 'serial child killers'". Sydney Morning Herald. Reuters. January 12, 2007.

50. Anne Bannon; Stevens, Serita Deborah (2007). *The Howdunit Book of Poisons (Howdunit)*. Cincinnati: Writers Digest Books. ISBN 1-58297-456-X.

51. "Truth Serums". *Television Tropes & Idioms*. Retrieved 27 July 2012.

52 Pearlman, T. (1980). "Behavioral desensitization of phobic anxiety using thiopental sodium". *The American Journal of Psychiatry* (American Psychiatric Association) **137** (12): 1580–1582. PMID 6108082.

53."Drugged Future?". *TIME*. February 24, 1958.

54. Snelders, Stephen (1998). "The LSD Therapy Career of Jan Bastiaans, M.D".*Newsletter of the Multidisciplinary Association for Psychedelic Studies* (Multidisciplinary Association for Psychedelic Studies) **8** (1): 18–20.

55. Weber, M; Motin, L; Gaul, S; Beker, F; Fink, RH; Adams, DJ (January 2005)."Intravenous anesthetics inhibit nicotinic acetyl-choline receptor-mediated currents and Ca2+ transients in rat intracardiac ganglion neurons". *British Journal of Pharmacology***144** (1): 98–107.

56. Franks, NP; Lieb, WR (23 November 1998). "Which molecular targets are most relevant to general anaesthesia?". *Toxicology Letters*. 100–101 (1–2): 1–8. doi:10.1016/S0378-4274(98)00158-1. PMID 10049127.

57. "Anesthesia and Analgesia". University of Virginia School of Medicine. Retrieved2007-08-05.

58. McKinley, Jesse (28 September 2010). "Judges Question California's Motivation on Execution". *New York Times*.

59 "U.S. Drug Maker Discontinues Key Death Penalty Drug". Fox News. 21 January 2011.

60. WINTERS WD, SPECTOR E, WALLACH DP, SHIDEMAN FE (July 1955). "Metabolism of thiopental-S35 and thiopental-2-C14 by a rat liver mince and identification of pentobarbital as a major metabolite". *J. Pharmacol. Exp. Ther.* **114** (3): 343–57. PMID 13243246. Retrieved 2008-07-18.[

61. Bory C; Chantin C; Boulieu R et al. (1986). "[Use of thiopental in man. Determination of this drug and its metabolites in plasma and urine by liquid phase chromatography and mass spectrometry]". *C. R. Acad. Sci. III, Sci. Vie* (in French) **303** (1): 7–12.PMID 3093002.

62. "Pentothal (thiopental)". eMedicineHealth. April 12, 2009.

63. M. F. M. James; R. J. Hift (July 1, 2000). "Porphyrias". *bja.oxfordjournals.org*. Retrieved September 25, 2013.

64. Pereda J; Gómez-Cambronero L; Alberola A et al. (October 2006). "Co-administration of pentoxifylline and thiopental causes death by acute pulmonary oedema in rats". *Br. J. Pharmacol.* **149** (4): 450–5. doi:10.1038/sj.bjp.0706871. PMC 1978439.PMID 16953192.

65. "This Month in Anesthesia History: March". Anesthesia History Association.

66. Steinhaus, John E (September 2001). "The Investigator and His 'Uncompromising Scientific Honesty'". *Asa Newsletter* (American Society of Anesthesiologists) **65** (9): 7–9.

67. Lundy, John S. (1966). "From this point in time: Some memories of my part in the history of anesthesia". *Journal of the American Association of Nurse Anesthetists* (American Association of Nurse Anesthetists) **24** (2): 95–102.

.

**68** Thatcher, Virginia S. (1953). "Chapter 7: Illegal or Legal?". *History of Anesthesia with Emphasis on the Nurse Specialist*. J.B. Lippincott. ISBN 0-8240-6525-5.

**69.** Bennetts FE (September 1995). "Thiopentone anaesthesia at Pearl Harbor". *Br J Anaesth* **75** (3): 366–8. doi:10.1093/bja/75.3.366. PMID 7547061. Retrieved2008-07-18.

70. Sachs HC and the American Academy of Pediatrics committee on Drugs. The transfer of drugs and therapeutics into human breast milk: An update on selected topics. Pediatrics. 2013;132:e796-809.

71. Baselt RC. Disposition of toxic drugs and chemicals in man. 6th ed. Foster City: Biomedical Publications, 2002:787-9.

72. Pokela ML, Anttila E, Seppala T et al. Marked variation in oxycodone pharmacokinetics in infants. Paediatr Anaesth. 2005;15:560-5. PMID: 15960639

73. Marx CM, Pucino F, Carlson JD et al. Oxycodone excretion in human milk in the puerperium. Drug Intell Clin Pharm. 1986;20:474. Abstract.

74. Seaton S, Reeves M, McLean S. Oxycodone as a component of multimodal analgesia for lactating mothers after Caesarean section: Relationships between maternal plasma, breast milk and neonatal plasma levels. Aust N Z J Obstet Gynaecol. 2007;47:181-5. PMID: 17550483

75. Sulton-Villavasso C, Austin CA, Patra KP et al. Index of suspicion. Case 1: Infant who has respiratory distress. Case 2: Abnormal behavior, seizures, and altered sensorium in a 7-year-old boy. Case 3: Fever and dysphagia in a 4-year-old girl. Pediatr Rev. 2012;33:279-84. PMID:22659261

76. Levine B, Moore KA, Aronica-Pollak P et al. Oxycodone intoxication in an infant: accidental or intentional exposure? J Forensic Sci. 2004;49:1358-60. PMID: 15568714

77. Rampono J, Kristensen JH, Ilett KF, Hackett LP, Kohan R. Quetiapine and breast feeding. Ann Pharmacother. 2007;41:711-4. PMID: 17374621

78. Lam J, Kelly L, Ciszkowski C et al. Central nervous system depression of neonates breastfed by mothers receiving oxycodone for postpartum analgesia. J Pediatr. 2012;160:33-37.e2. PMID:21880331

79. Timm NL. Maternal use of oxycodone resulting in opioid intoxication in her breastfed neonate. J Pediatr. 2013;162:421-2. PMID: 23063265

80. Saarialho-Kere U, Mattila MJ, Seppala T. Psychomotor, respiratory and neuroendocrinological effects of a mu-opioid receptor agonist (oxycodone) in healthy volunteers. Pharmacol Toxicol. 1989;65:252-7. PMID: 2555803

81. Esener Z, Sarihasan B, Guven H et al. Thiopentone and etomidate concentrations in maternal and umbilical plasma, and in colostrum. Br J Anaesth. 1992;69:586-8.

82. Borgatta L, Jenny RW, Gruss L et al. Clinical significance of methohexital, meperidine, and diazepam in breast milk. J Clin Pharmacol. 1997;37:186-92.

83. Edwards JE, Rudy AC, Wermeling DP et al. Hydromorphone transfer into breast milk after intranasal administration. Pharmacotherapy. 2003;23:153-8.

84. Tolis G, Dent R, Guyda H. Opiates, prolactin, and the dopamine receptor. J Clin Endocrinol Metab. 1978;47:200-3.

85. Fang et al. (1995). "Carbon Monoxide Production from Degradation of Desflurane". Anesthesia and Analgesia.

**86.** Sulbaek Andersen MP, Sander SP, Nielsen OJ, Wagner DS, Sanford Jr TJ, Wallington TJ (July 2010). "Inhalation anaesthetics and climate change". *British Journal of Anaesthesia* **105** (6): 760–766. doi:10.1093/bja/aeq259.

**87.** *Anesthesia & Analgesia* (San Francisco, CA:International Anesthesia Research Society) **111** (1): 92–98.doi:10.1213/ane.0b013e3181e058d7. Retrieved 9 September 2011.

**88.** Ryan SM, Nielsen CJ (July 2010). "Global Warming Potential of Inhaled Anesthetics: Application to Clinical Use". *Anesthesia and Analgesia* **111** (1): 92–98.doi:10.1213/ane.0b013e3181e058d7.

**89.** Kim JK (Feb 2014). "Relationship of bispectral index to minimum alveolar concentration during isoflurane, sevoflurane or desflurane anaesthesia.". *J Int Med Res* **42** (1): 130–7

90. Berlin CM Jr, Yaffe SJ, Ragni M. Disposition of acetaminophen in milk, saliva and plasma of lactating women. Pediatr Pharmacol. 1980;1:135-41.

91. Bitzen PO, Gustafsson B, Jostell KG et al. Excretion of paracetamol in human breast milk. Eur J Clin Pharmacol. 1981;20:123-5.

92. Notarianni LJ, Oldham HG, Bennett PN. Passage of paracetamol into breast milk and its subsequent metabolism by the neonate. Br J Clin Pharmacol. 1987;24:63-7

93. Matheson I, Lunde PKM, Notarianni L. Infant rash caused by paracetamol in breast milk? Pediatrics. 1985;76:651-2. Letter.

94. Findlay JWA, DeAngelis RL et al. Analgesic drugs in breast milk and plasma. Clin Pharmacol Ther. 1981;29:625-33.

95. Ito S, Blajchman A, Stephenson M et al. Prospective follow-up of adverse reactions in breast-fed infants exposed to maternal medication. Am J Obstet Gynecol. 1993;168:1393-9

96. Nadal-Amat J , Verd S. Paracetamol and asthma and lactation. Acta Paediatr. 2011;100:e2-3

97. Bakkeheim E, Carlsen KH, Lodrup Carlsen KC. Paracetamol exposure during breastfeeding and risk of allergic disease. Acta Paediatr. 2011;100:e3. PMID: 21535130

98. Pittman KA, Smyth RD, Losada M et al. Human perinatal distribution of butorphanol. Am J Obstet Gynecol. 1980;138 (7 Pt 1):797-800.

99. Tolis G, Dent R, Guyda H. Opiates, prolactin, and the dopamine receptor. J Clin Endocrinol Metab. 1978;47:200-3.

100. Saarialho-Kere U. Psychomotor, respiratory and neuroendocrinological effects of nalbuphine and haloperidol, alone and in combination, in healthy subjects. Br J Clin Pharmacol. 1988;26:79-87.

101. Crowell MK, Hill PD, Humenick SS. Relationship between obstetric analgesia and time of effective breast feeding. J Nurse Midwifery. 1994;39:150-6.

102. Lind JN, Perrine CG, Li R. Relationship between use of labor pain medications and delayed onset of lactation. J Hum Lact. 2014;30:167-73.

103. Jamali F, Tam YK, Stevens RD. Naproxen excretion in breast milk and its uptake by suckling infant. Drug Intell Clin Pharm. 1982;16:475. Abstract.

104. Jamali F, Stevens DR. Naproxen excretion in milk and its uptake by the infant. Drug Intell Clin Pharm. 1983;17:910-1.

105. Fidalgo I, Correa R, Gomez Carrasco JA et al. [Acute anemia, rectorrhagia and hematuria caused by ingestion of naproxen]. An Esp Pediatr. 1989;30:317-9.

106. Ito S, Blajchman A, Stephenson M et al. Prospective follow-up of adverse reactions in breast-fed infants exposed to maternal medication. Am J Obstet Gynecol. 1993;168:1393-9.

107. Sammour RN, Ohel G, Cohen M, Gonen R. Oral naproxen versus oral tramadol for analgesia after cesarean delivery. Int J Gynaecol Obstet. 2011;113:144-7.

108. Weibert RT, Townsend RJ, Kaiser DG et al. Lack of ibuprofen secretion into human milk. Clin Pharm. 1982;1:457-8.

109. Townsend RJ, Benedetti TJ, Erickson SH et al. Excretion of ibuprofen into breast milk. Am J Obstet Gynecol. 1984;149:184-6.

110. Walter K, Dilger C. Ibuprofen in human milk. Br J Clin Pharmacol. 1997;44:211-2.

111. Rigourd V, de Villepin B, Amirouche A et al. Ibuprofen concentrations in human mature milk-First data about pharmacokinetics study in breast milk with AOR-10127 "Antalait" study. Ther Drug Monit. 2014;36:590-6.

112. Ito S, Blajchman A, Stephenson M. Prospective follow-up of adverse reactions in breast-fed infants exposed to maternal medication. Am J Obstet Gynecol. 1993;168:1393-9

113. Cox SR, Forbes KK. Excretion of flurbiprofen into breast milk. Pharmacotherapy. 1987;7:211-5

114. Smith IJ, Hinson JL, Johnson VA et al. Flurbiprofen in post-partum women: plasma and breast milk disposition. J Clin Pharmacol. 1989;29:174-84.

115. Ostensen M. Piroxicam in human breast milk. Eur J Clin Pharmacol. 1983;25:829-30

116. Ostensen M, Matheson I, Laufen H. Piroxicam in breast milk after long-term treatment. Eur J Clin Pharmacol. 1988;35:567-9. 117. 118.

117.Lebedevs TH, Wojnar-Horton RE, Yapp P et al. Excretion of indomethacin in breast milk. Br J Clin Pharmacol. 1991;32:751-4.

118. Beaulac-Baillargeon L, Allard G. Distribution of indomethacin in human milk and estimation of its milk to plasma ratio in vitro. Br J Clin Pharmacol. 1993;36:413-6

119. Eeg-Olofsson O, Malmros I, Elwin CE, Steen B. Convulsions in a breast-fed infant after maternal indomethacin. Lancet. 1978;2 (8082):215. Letter.

## Book references and Additional Reading

- Eger, Eisenkraft, Weiskopf. The Pharmacology of Inhaled Anesthetics. 2003.
- Rang, Dale, Ritter, Moore. Pharmacology 5th Edition. 2003.
- Martin Bellgardt: Evaluation der Sedierungstiefe und der Aufwachzeiten frisch operierter Patienten mit neurophysiologischem Monitoring im Rahmen der Studie: Desfluran versus Propofol zur Sedierung beatmeter Patienten. Bochum, Dissertation, 2005 (pdf)
- Susanne Lohmann: Verträglichkeit, Nebenwirkungen und Hämodynamik der inhalativen Sedierung mit Desfluran im Rahmen der Studie: Desfluran versus
- Propofol zur Sedierung beatmeter Patienten. Bochum, Dissertation, 2006 (pdf)

Patel SS, Goa KL. (1995) "Desflurane. A review of its pharmacodynamic and pharmacokinetic properties and its efficacy in general anaesthesia." Drugs Oct;50(4):742-67.PMID 8536556.

**Research article;**

**Comparison between the effect of total intravenous anesthesia (TIVA), and sevoflurane based anesthesia (VIMA), on breast feeding lactation.**

Authers: Hala Mostafa Goma, professor of anesthesia, faculty of medicine Cairo University Egypt

Corresponding author Hala Mostafa assistant professor of anesthesia faculty of medicine Cairo University,Egypt.

Ahmeda1995@ yahoo.com

**Abstract:**

**objectives**: *Breast feeding behavior of infants* may be affected when Lactating mothers were exposed to anesthetic agents, it is very important for the anesthetic drugs to be of short half life and has less metabolites that can be transmitted to the baby via breast milk. Aim of this study is to compare sevoflurane and propofol effects on infant's breast feeding behavior.Patients and methods: the study was Prospective, cross-sectional, comparative study.

This study was conducted on 20 lactating women underwent ≤one hour surgical procedures. They were divided in two groups .Group 1 (n=10) received sevoflurane in the induction, and maintenance of anesthesia .Group 2 (n=10) received propofol in the induction, and maintenance of anesthesia. Parameters measured were infants feeding behavior score for both groups at 2, 4, 6,12hours postoperatively.*Results:* Infants had rooting reflex 2 (80%) in sevoflurane group while (30%) in propofol group. nipple grasps score 3 (40%) in sevoflurane group while (10%) in propofol group. swallowing reflex score 2 (60%) in sevoflurane group while (20%) in propofol group. Total score was 10-12  and 8-10 in sevoflurane and propofol respectively  P value <0.001. Duration of each meal in minutes was 2.4(0.5) in sevoflurane group and 2.00 (0.00).

Conclusion:

The study concluded that both sevoflurane and propofol have accepted infant's breastfeeding score, but sevoflurane had a significant higher score than propofol.

Key words:

Breast feeding behavior, propofol, sevoflurane

## Introduction:

Breast milk is considered the ideal nutrition for infants. Early contact is essential for initiation of breast feeding; American Academy of Pediatrics recommends that, whenever possible, breast milk be the only milk that infants receive for the first year (1). , in addition to the psychological relationships between mothers and babies, breast milk is essential for the immune system, a nutritionally complete food source with low cost. There are many factors that may affect initiation of breast feeding, *mother factors* as the multiparty, regularity of breast feeding, the use of supplemental bottle feeding, ethnic status of the mother, the socioeconomic status, and other maternal factors such as inverted nipples, lack of education, or incentive. *Infants' issues* as the infant cannot latch onto the breast or suckle well, the presence of palatal structure abnormalities, or the presence of congenital neurological abnormalities (2). Mothers exposed to anesthetic drugs during general anesthesia which may affect lactation, besides the operative pain that may also suppress lactation (3). It is very important to choose anesthetic drugs which have short half life and has less metabolite that can be transmitted to the baby via breast milk. Most of the studies compared the effects of the drugs specially the narcotics when used epidurally or intrathecally on early breast feeding (4).

There are little studies compared the effects of general anesthetics on breast feeding behavior of infants. Sevoflurane is an inhaled general anesthetic, which has low blood – gas coefficient, so it has rapid induction and recovery time (5). Propofol is a 2,6-diisopropylphenol with sedative-hypnotic properties, so it has also rapid induction and recovery time (6).

The aim of this study is to compare the effects of sevoflurane and propofol when used as maintenance drugs during general anesthesia and the breast feeding behaviors of infants.

### *Patients and methods:*

After patients written consents ,a  prospective comparative randomized study was conducted, 20 lactating mothers scheduled for elective surgical procedures under general anesthesia in kasr El AIni teaching hospital; they were divided in 2 groups each group 10 patients.

 inclusion criteria were, age  20-40 years, all mothers are healthy multipara who gave birth to full term healthy newborns,  surgical procedures were ≤1 hour.

Exclusion criteria, any history of breast feeding problems for both mothers and infants, supplemented bottle lactation.

Routine monitoring was by using ECG, noninvasive blood pressure, pulse oximeter, capnography. No premedication was given.

In group 1 Induction was achieved by using sevoflurane by face mask with 6 liter 100% Oxygen, the concentration of sevoflurane was 0.5% and increased gradually to reach 4%. In group 2 induction was achieved by using propofol 1-2mg/kg IV, 100% oxygen via face mask. 1 µg/kg fentanyl was given to all studied patients.

Signs of complete induction of anesthesia were absence of eye lash reflex, absence of the response for verbal command, absence of movement, coughing, tearing, increased heart rate and blood pressure more than 15% from the base line.

Atracurium 0.4 mg/kg IV was given for intubation in all patients. Cuffed endotracheal tubes were used. Ventilation rate was 10 per minute, and the tidal volume was 6-8 ml /kg, end tidal $CO_2$ was maintained between 30-35 mmHg.

Maintenance of anesthesia was achieved by using 2%sevoflurane with 3 liter/min 70% oxygen in air in group 1.

In group 2 anesthesias was maintained by using propofol IV infusion at a rate of 50-150µ/kg/min, muscle relaxation was maintained   by0.05 mg/kg atracurium in all patients.

At the end of surgical procedures Reversal of muscle relaxant was achieved by using 0.06 mg/kg neostigmine and 0.1 mg/kg atropine.

Postoperative analgesia was conducted with local infiltration of lidocaine 2% in the operative site, paracetamol IV infusion (Perflgan ), narcotics were avoided .

Assessment of the infant *(breast feeding Behavior* score ) (7) was done by a pediatric consultant . Parameters were assessed were (rooting reflex, nipple grasp, duration of the each meal, strength of suckling and swallowing and the total of 14) .The parameters were assessed at 2,4,6,8,10,12 hours postoperatively. .

**Rooting reflex.**

| | |
|---|---|
| **Did not root** | **0** |
| **Showed some rooting behavior** | **1** |
| **Showed obvious rooting behavior** | **2** |

**Areolar grasp .**

| | |
|---|---|
| **Non,the mouth only touched the nipple** | **0** |
| **Part of the nipple** | **1** |
| **The whole nipple not areola** | **2** |
| **The nipple and some the areola** | **3** |

**Suckling.**

| | |
|---|---|
| No suckling | 0 |
| Licking and tasting but not suckling | 1 |
| single suckling | 2 |
| Repeated short suckling (Less than 10) | 3 |
| Repeated more than 2 long burst | 4 |

**Swallowing.**

| | |
|---|---|
| Was not noticed | 0 |
| Occasional swallowing was noticed | 1 |
| Repeated swallowing was noticed | 2 |

| Duration of the meal. | | |
|---|---|---|
| Did not latch at all | 0 | |
| Latched for 5 minutes | 1 | |
| Latched 6-10 minutes | 2 | |
| Latched 11-15 minutes | 3 | |
| Total score | 14 | (7) |

Statistical analysis : data were represented as mean(SD) analysis was done by using SPSS version 15, T-test and Chi-square test.

*p≤0.05 is considered significant.

*Results:*

## Table 1:Demographic data of the both groups:

| | Group1 (sevoflurane group) (n=10) | Group2 (propofol group) (n=10) |
|---|---|---|
| Age(yr) | 28.6(7.3) | 30.8(7.7) |
| Weight(kg) | 80.3(7.7) | 89.8(9.3) |
| Height(cm) | 167.7(7.3) | 170.9(8.3) |

Table 1 shows no significant difference in age, weight and height of both groups.

*p≤0.05 is considered significant.

**Table 2: Rooting reflex score in both groups.**

| Rooting reflex score | Group1 (sevoflurane group) (n=10) | Group2 (propofol group) (n=10) |
|---|---|---|
| 1 | 4(20%) | 14(70%)* |
| 2 | 16(80%)* | 6(30%) |

Infants had rooting reflex 2 (80%) in sevoflurane group while (30%) in propofol group.

Rooting reflex is significantly higher in sevoflurane group than propofol group.

P value = 0.001.

*p≤0.05 is considered significant.

**Table 3: nipple grasps score in both groups.**

| Nipple grasp score | Group1 | group 2 |
|---|---|---|
| 2 | 12(60%) | 18(90%) |
| 3 | 8(40%)* | 2(10%) |

Infants had nipple grasps score 3 (40%) in sevoflurane group while
(10%) in propofol group.

Nipple grasps score is significantly higher in sevoflurane group than
in propofol group.

P value 0.028

*p≤0.05 is considered significant.

**Table 4: swallowing reflex score in both groups.**

| Swallowing reflex score | Group1 | Group 2 ) |
|---|---|---|
| 1 | 8(40%) | 16(80%) |
| 2 | 12(60%) | 4(20%) |
| P value | 0.010 | |

Infants had swallowing reflex score 2 (60%) in sevoflurane group while (20%) in propofol group.

Swallowing reflex score is significantly higher in sevoflurane group than in propofol group.

P value 0.010

*p≤0.05 is considered significant.

**Table 5:Duration of each meal in minutes and the total score:**

|  | Group1 | group 2 |
|---|---|---|
| Duration of each meal in minutes | 2.4(0.5)* | 2.00(0.00) |
| Total score | 10-12 | 8-10 |

Table 5:Duration of meals are significantly longer in sevoflurane group than propofol group p value =0.002

*p≤0.05 is considered significant.

**Table 6:  strength of suckling score.**

| Score of strength of suckling | Group1 (sevoflurane group) (n=20) | group 2 (propofol group) (n=20) |
|---|---|---|

| | | |
|---|---|---|
| 2 | 0(0%) | 8(40%)* |
| 3 | 8(40%) | 12(60%)* |
| 4 | 12(60%) * | 0(0%) |

Strength of suckling score 4 (60 %) in group 1 while 0 in group 2.

Strength of suckling score 3 (40% in group 1 while 60% in group 2.

Strength of suckling was significantly higher in sevoflurane group than propofol group P value<0.001.

*p≤0.05 is considered significant.

## Discussion:

Breast feeding is very important for both mothers and infants, according to American academy recommend breast milk lactation in the first year of life (1). Mothers may be exposed to general anesthesia during the period of lactation .There is no sufficient data about the effect of anesthetic drugs on human lactation.

Many studies conducted on the effects of anesthesia on breast lactation, they gave a great concern about the effects of narcotics in epidural and general anesthesia during cesarean section. They demonstrated the gain of the early  eye and skin contact between mothers and infants on initiation of lactation (8). Some studies determined the level of narcotics in colostrum after high dose of epidural fentanyl ( 9). Other studies demonstrated the relation between type of anesthesia and the continuation of breast feeding lactation after surgical procedures (10). American academy recommended the short acting and easily  eliminated drug with the minimum dose should be used (1).  The mothers should weigh the benefit of continuation of lactation against the effect of anesthetics on infants. However the WHO listed anesthetic drugs that can be safely used during lactation (12). There is no sufficient data about some

Anesthetics as sevoflurane and propofol, and which is better to be used .The present study compared sevoflurane and propofol on breast feeding behavior. The study found that breast feeding score was significantly higher in sevoflurane than propofol group. The explanation may be that sevoflurane, a potent inhalational anesthetic with a blood-gas partition coefficient of 0.60, provides a relatively rapid inhalation induction and recovery from anesthesia, the low coefficient facilitate its elimination via the lungs. Binding of sevoflurane to blood protein is not yet investigated. It is metabolized by cytochrom P 450 to Hexfluroisopropranol, fluoride and $CO_2$. Hexfluroisopropranol conjugated in the liver and eliminated by the kidney (5). On the other hand, Propofol is a highly protein-bound drug and is metabolized by conjugation in the liver. Its rate of clearance exceeds hepatic blood flow, suggesting an extra hepatic site of elimination as well. Propofol is rapidly distributed into peripheral tissues so; it has short duration of action. The half life of elimination of propofol is 2 - 24 hours (6).Limitation of the study that it was only for 12 hours while it needs to be more, at least 24 hours, but because of the ethical point of view the study time is shorter.

The study concluded that both sevoflurane and propofol are short acting drugs and both have good breast feeding score, but sevoflurane has a significant higher score than propofol. There is no sufficient data about the level of sevoflurane or its metabolites (Hexfluroisopropranol, fluoride) in the breast milk. More studies are recommended to compare the level of sevoflurane and propofol and their metabolites in breast milk.

**References:**

1. American Academy of Pediatrics, Committee on Drugs.(2001): The transfer of drugs and other chemicals into human milk. Pediatrics, 108(3), 776–789.

.2.Beilin, Y., Bodian, C. A., Weiser, J., Hossain, S., Ittamar,A., Feierman, D., et al. (2005) : Effect of labor epidural analgesia with and without fentanyl on infant breast-feeding: A prospective, randomized, double blind study. Anesthesiology, 103(6), 1211–1217.

3. Briggs, G. G., Freeman, R. K., & Yaffe, S. J. (2005): Drugs in pregnancy and lactation (7th ed.). Philadelphia: Lippincott, Williams & Wilkins.

4. Dennis, C. L. (2002): Breastfeeding initiation and duration: A 1990–2000 literature review. Journal of Obstetric, Gynecologic, & Neonatal Nursing, 31(3), 247.

5. Ysuda N ,lockhart S ,Egar EL(1991): Comparison between isoflurane and sevoflurane in human .Anesthesia analgesia 72-316.

6.Nitsun M, Szokol JW, Saleh HJ, Murphy GS, Vender JS, Luong L, Raikoff K, Avram MJ(2006) : Pharmacokinetics of midazolam, propofol, and fentanyl transfer to human breast milk ,Clin Pharmacol Ther.; 79(6):549-57.

7. **Kerstin Hedberg Nyqvist, RN, MS** (1996): Development of the Preterm Infant Breast feeding Behavior Scale (PIBBS): A Study of Nurse-Mother Agreement.
Vol. 12, No. 3, 207-219.

8. McElhatton, P. R. (1994): The effects of benzodiazepine use during pregnancy and lactation. Reproductive Toxicology, 8(6), 461–475.

9. Spigset, O., & Hagg, S. (2000): Analgesics and breastfeeding: Safety considerations. Pediatric Drugs, 2(3).

10. Jensen D, Wallace S, Kelsay P. LATCH: a breast feeding charting system and documentation tool. J Obstet Gynecol Neonatal Nurs 1994;23:27–32.

11. Tsen, L. C. (2005): What's new and novel in obstetric anesthesia? Contributions from the 2003 scientific literature.
International Journal of Obstetric Anesthesia, 14,
126–146.

12. World Health Organization (2002): Breast feeding and maternal medication: Recommendations for drugs in the eleventh WHO Model list of essential drugs.

Retrieved May 12, 2006, from http://www.who.int/ child-adolescent-health/New_Publications/NUTRITION/BF_Maternal_Medication.pdf

WILLIAM HOWIE is a staff nurse anesthetist at the R.

www.ingramcontent.com/pod-product-compliance
Lightning Source LLC
Chambersburg PA
CBHW070909180526
45168CB00005B/1979